Camron & Isaiah Take on COVID

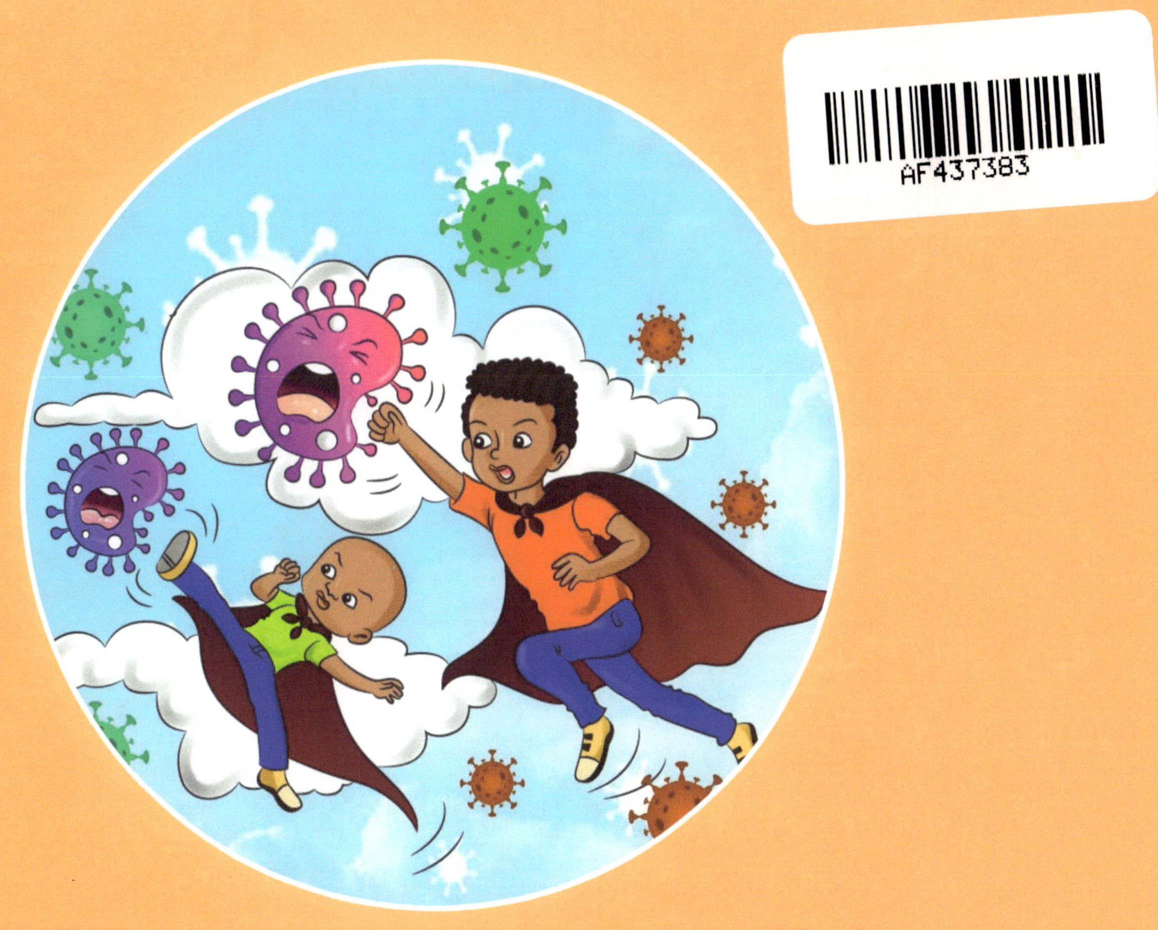

By: Deloshier Greene

I would like to dedicate this book to my amazing sons, Camron and Isaiah, my supportive husband, Desmine, all of my loveable nieces and nephews, my siblings, Shaloshier and Daren Jr.,my parents, Daren and Colette, and my spiritual parents Bishop Robertson and Co-Pastor Elena Robertson for the push I needed to get started. Last, but definitely not least, I thank you God for sending the Holy Spirit as a guide to help every step of the way.

On Thursday, March 12th we all went to school like a normal day. We didn't know that everything was about to change overnight.

"Bye, Mom. I love you" Camron said as he was leaving the house to catch the bus. "I love you, too" said Mom, as she was getting Isaiah dressed.

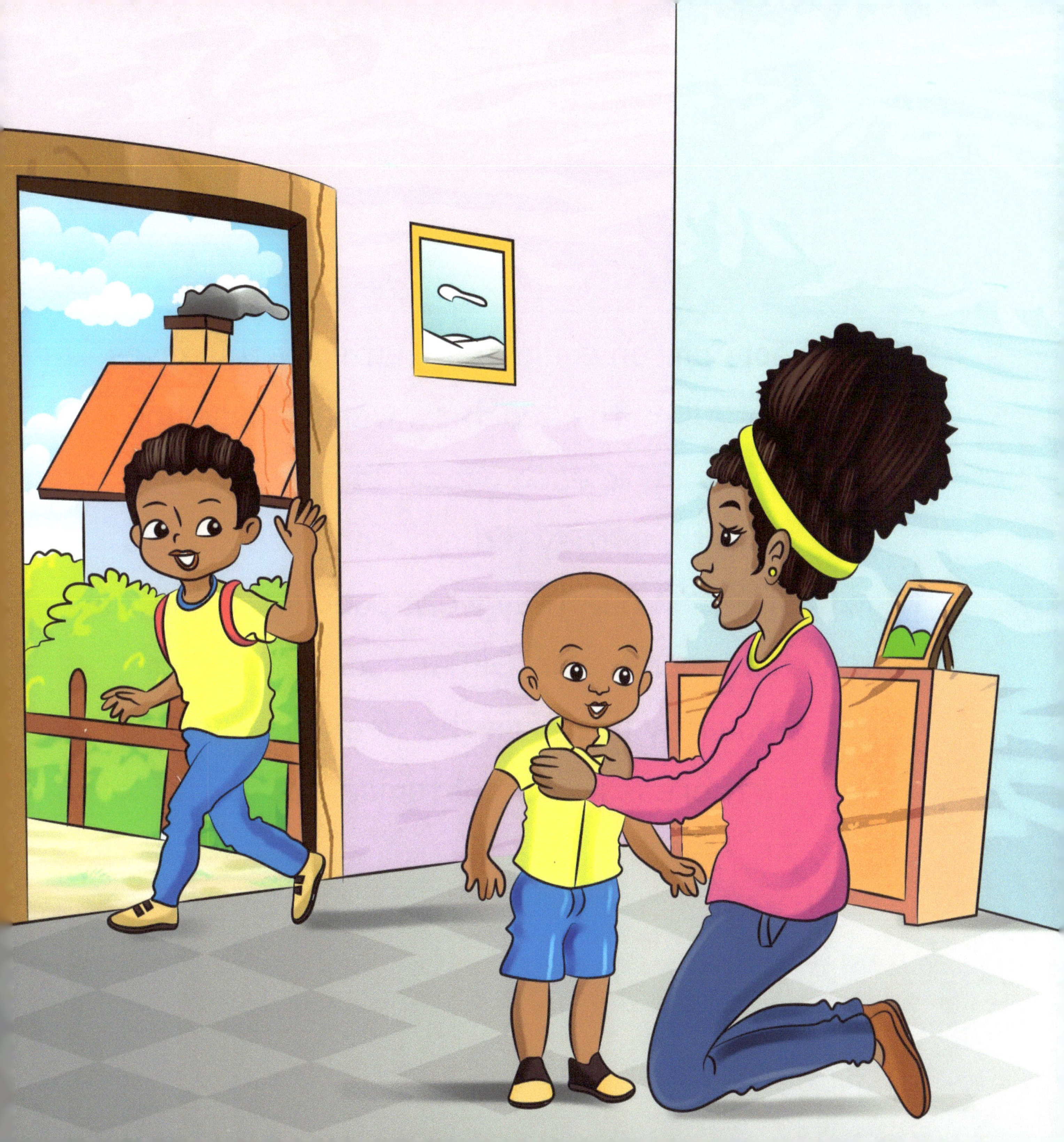

At school Camron could tell that something was going on. All of the teachers were whispering during the day to each other. It was like they knew something they did not want the kids to know just yet. While they were packing up for the day, his teacher, Mr. Gilbert said, "Get your things you may need for the weekend because there is no school tomorrow."

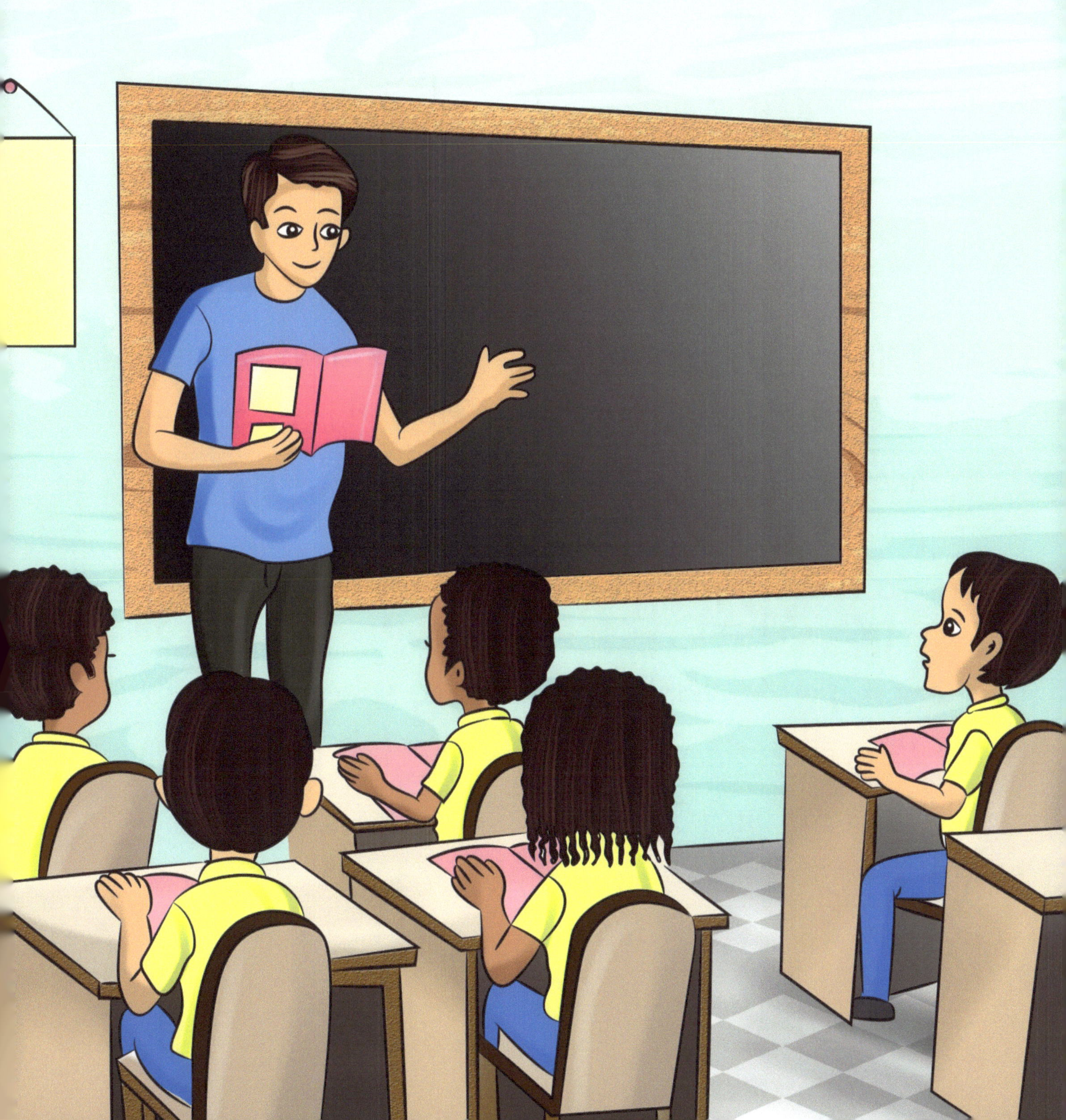

The whole classroom went into a roar of excitement. But, wait: there's not a holiday tomorrow. 'My mom would've told me if we didn't have school tomorrow, after all she is a teacher at another school,' Camron thought. 'Maybe this is a joke.'

"Mr. Gilbert", Camron said above the noise of excitement. "Why don't we have school tomorrow?" Mr. Gilbert said that he wasn't 100 percent sure but that our parents would get information soon. 'Weird,' Camron thought.

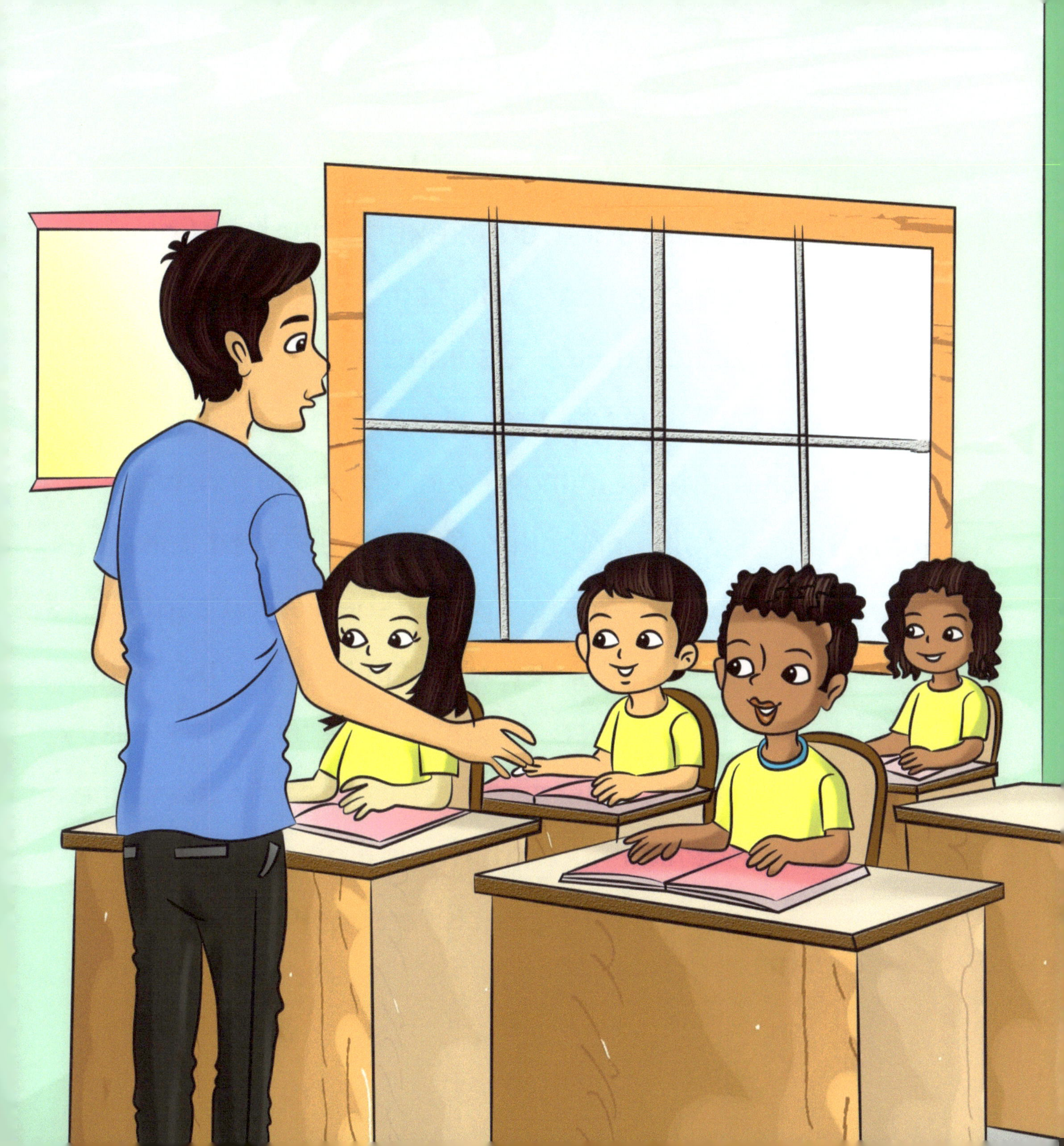

"Camron!!", Isaiah shouted in excitement as Camron walked through the door. "Hi, Isaiah," Camron said as he gave Isaiah a hug. "Isaiah I have no school tomorrow, but I don't know why," said Camron. They both looked at their mom, searching for answers. "Something is going on called COVID-19, also known as the Coronavirus," Mom started as she took a seat. "It's a virus that is making a lot of people sick, kind of like the flu but a little more dangerous because it's easily spread. The school district just wants to make sure everyone is safe and that the buildings are clean before we go back to school."

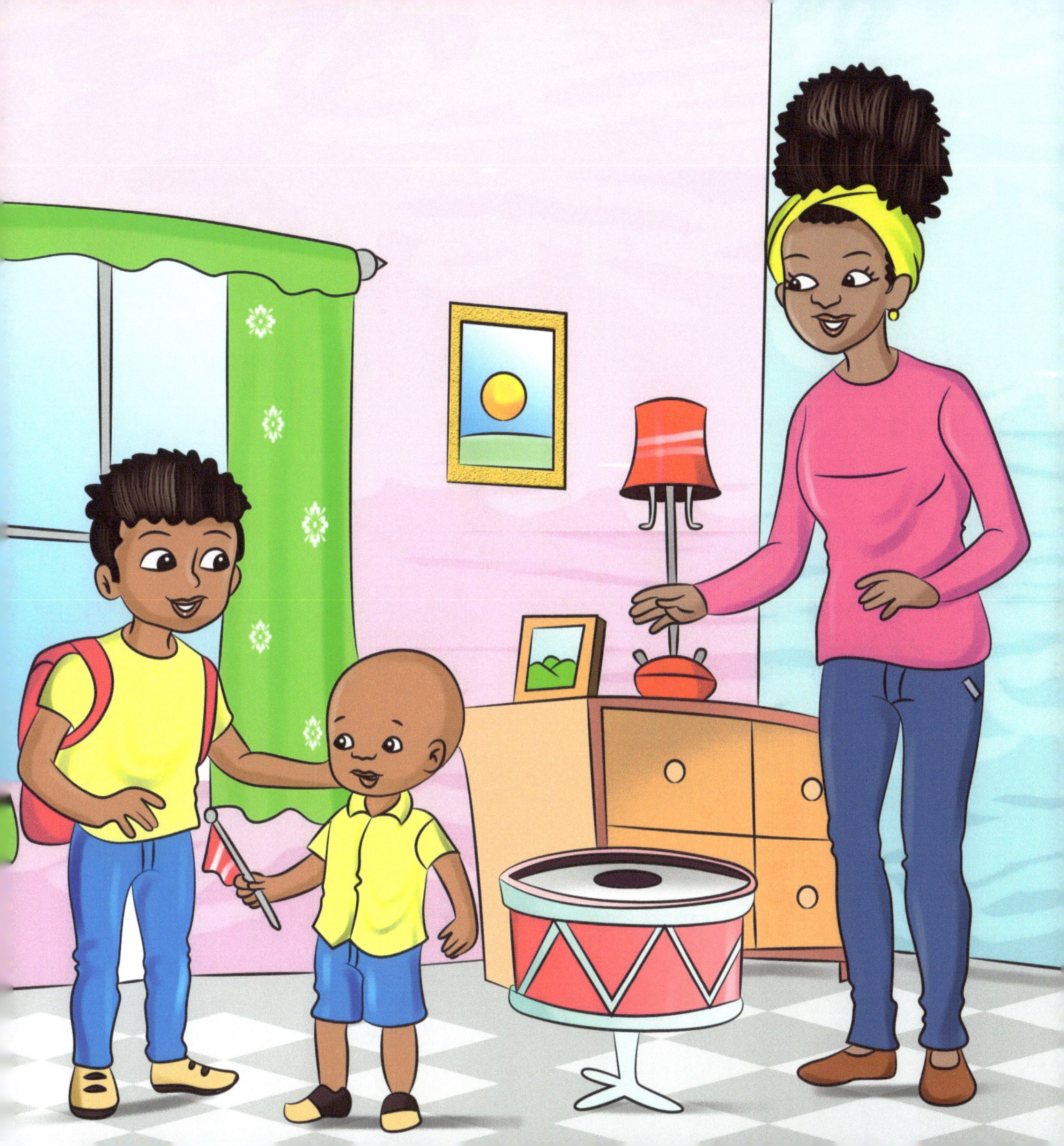

The next morning, when Camron and Isaiah wake up, their dad is still home. He is in the Army, so he always has to leave for work before they wake up. 'This is strange', Camron thought while also being happy to see his dad. "Daddy, you're off today?", Camron asked. "It looks like I'm going to be off for a while," began his dad. "We all are." Camron and Isaiah's parents explained that the coronavirus was something that no one, not even the really important scientists, knew anything about. It was affecting people all over the U.S. and even all over the world. They explained that everything was shutting down for the next two weeks and no one could go out unless it was for emergencies or unless they needed groceries.

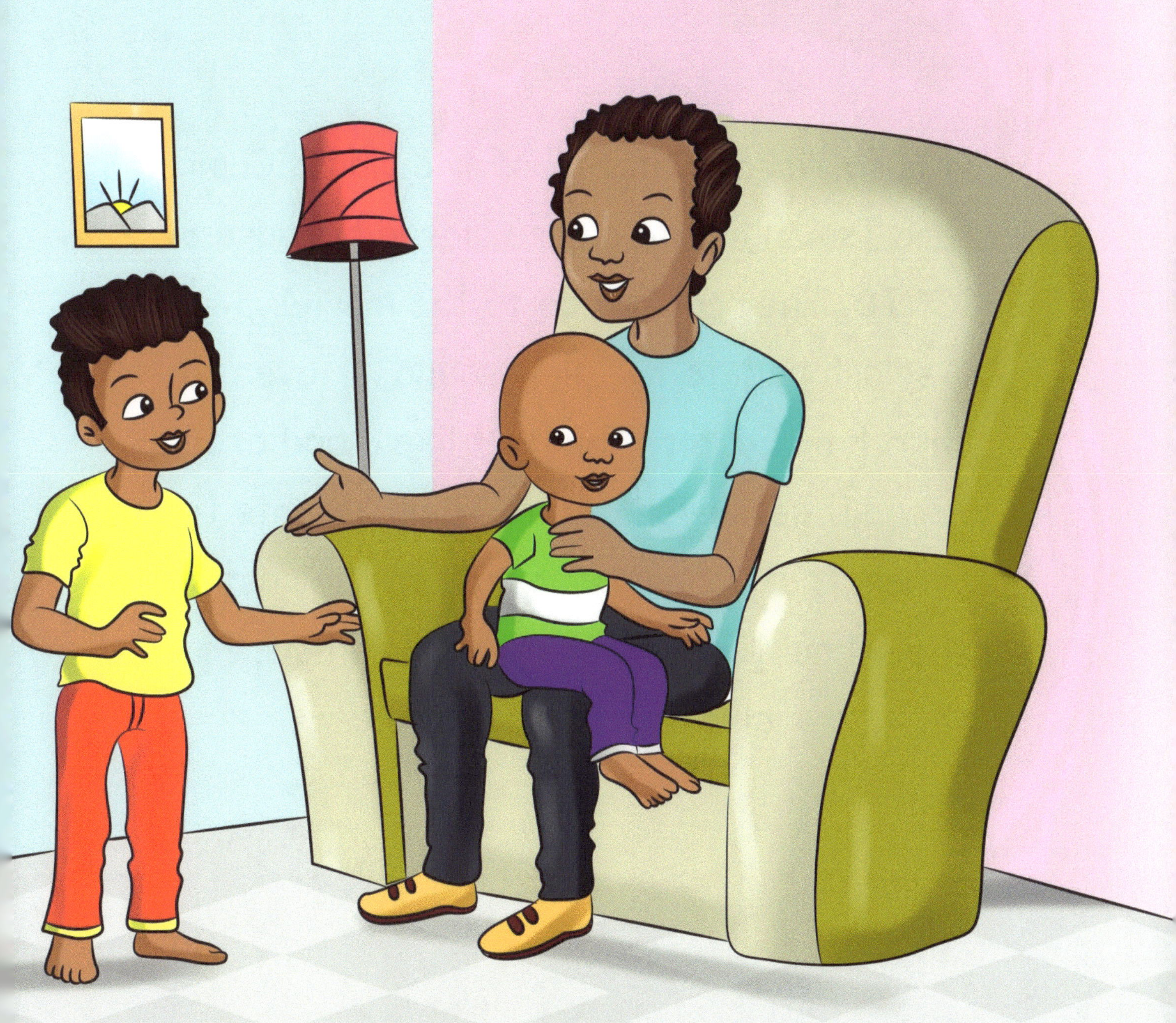

It is so strange that all of the places Camron and Isaiah like to go are closed because of COVID. They can not go to the movies, to the splash pad, to the playground, or even to church on Easter! This felt like a bad dream. Soon it gets even worse. Their parents tell them that school is closed for the rest of the school year and that they will have to do all of their work online.

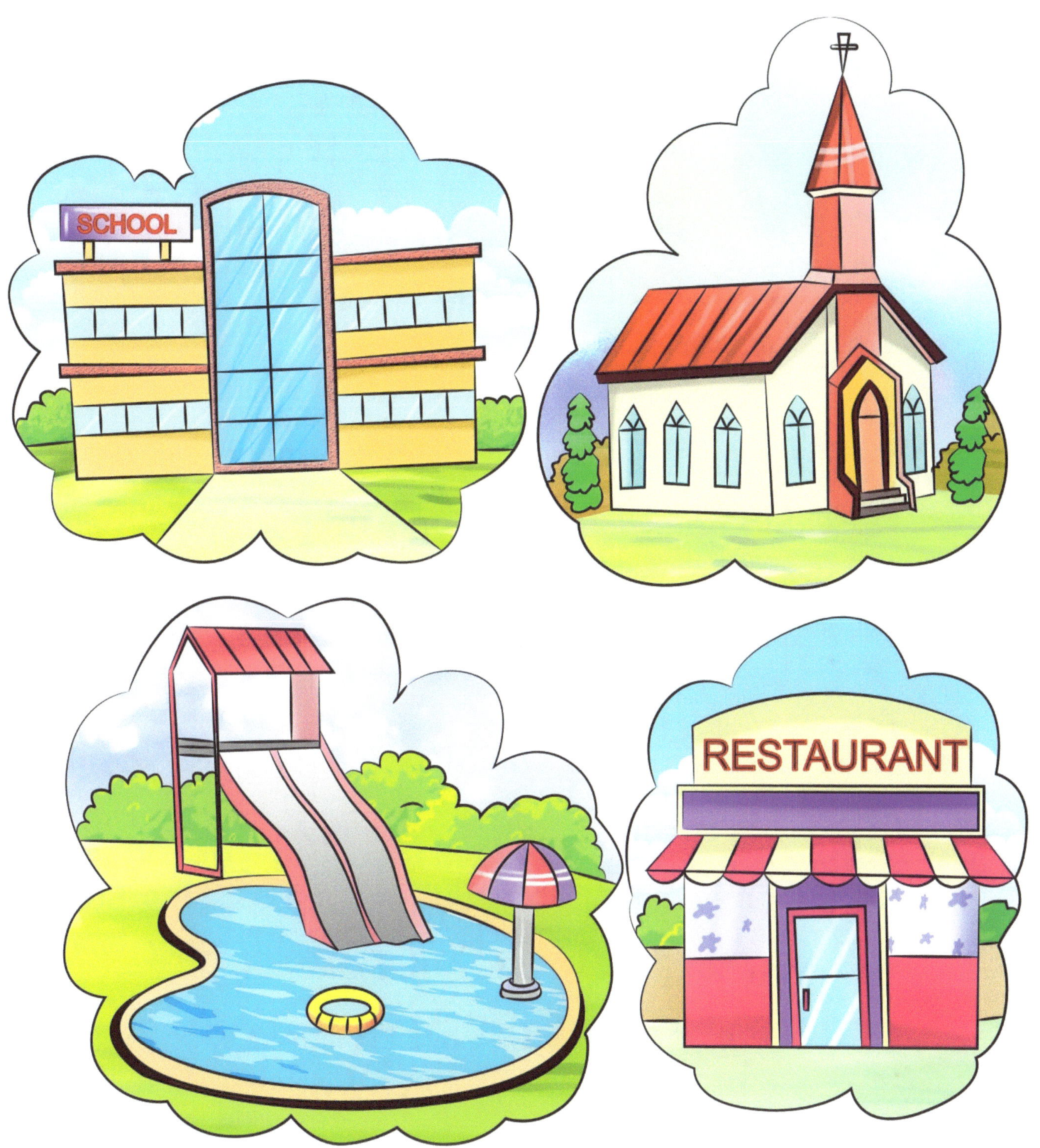

SCHOOL
RESTAURANT

It's fun to stay home for the first two weeks, but then things begin to get very boring. All of the sports are canceled on tv, and they still cannot go anywhere fun.

"Mom, I'm bored! This is not fun anymore. I wish COVID would go away!" Camron said pouting. "Me, too!" Isaiah whined. "I want to go to the playground."

"I know it's hard," began Mom as she hugged them. "But, COVID is being spread by simply coughing and spreading germs through touching things. It's not safe for you to go out now, but I promise we will have some fun while we're home".

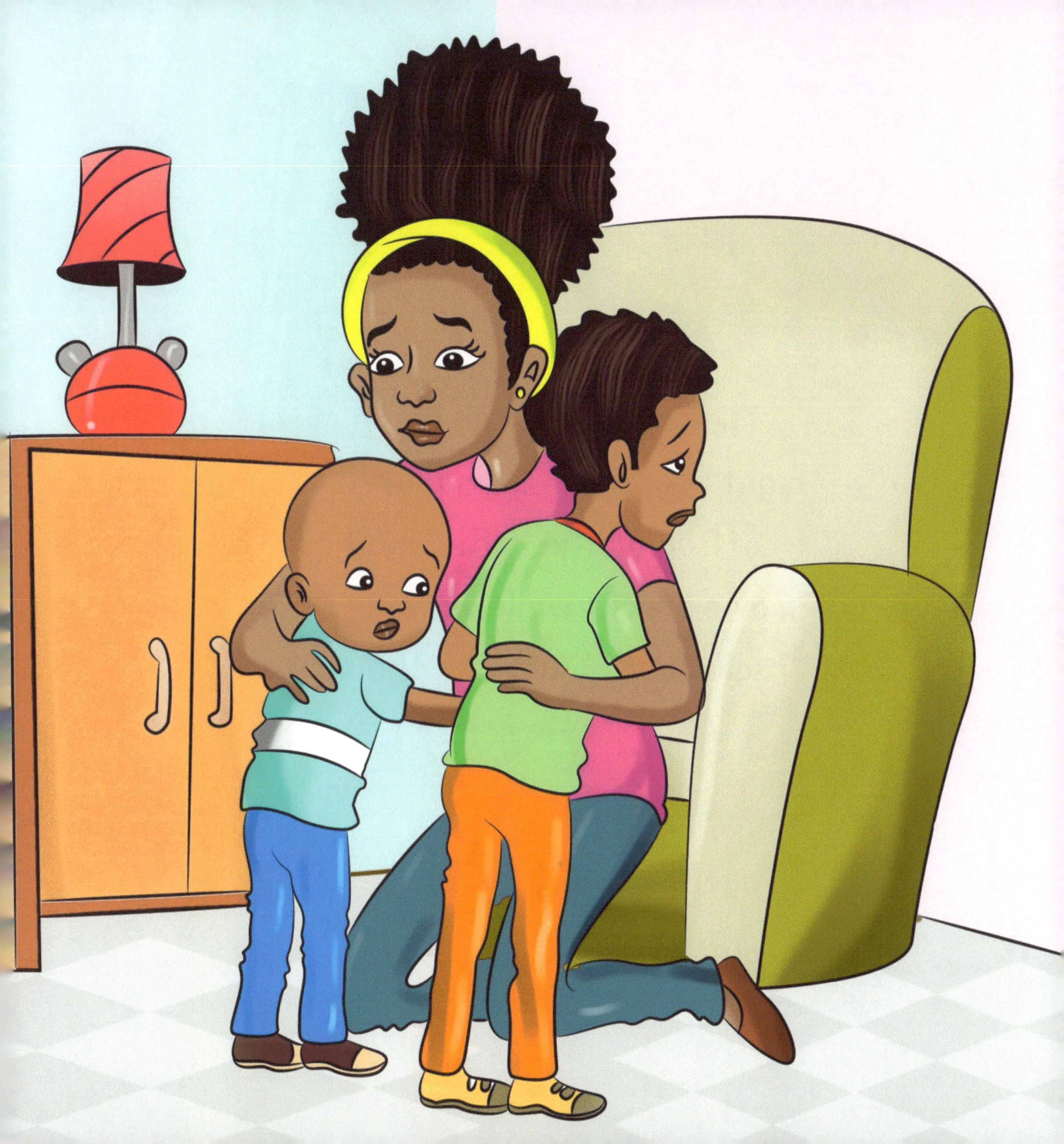

That night they all had a movie
night together. Isaiah loved turning
off all of the lights and having
movie snacks while watching the tv
really loud. "Just like the movies!"
He said.

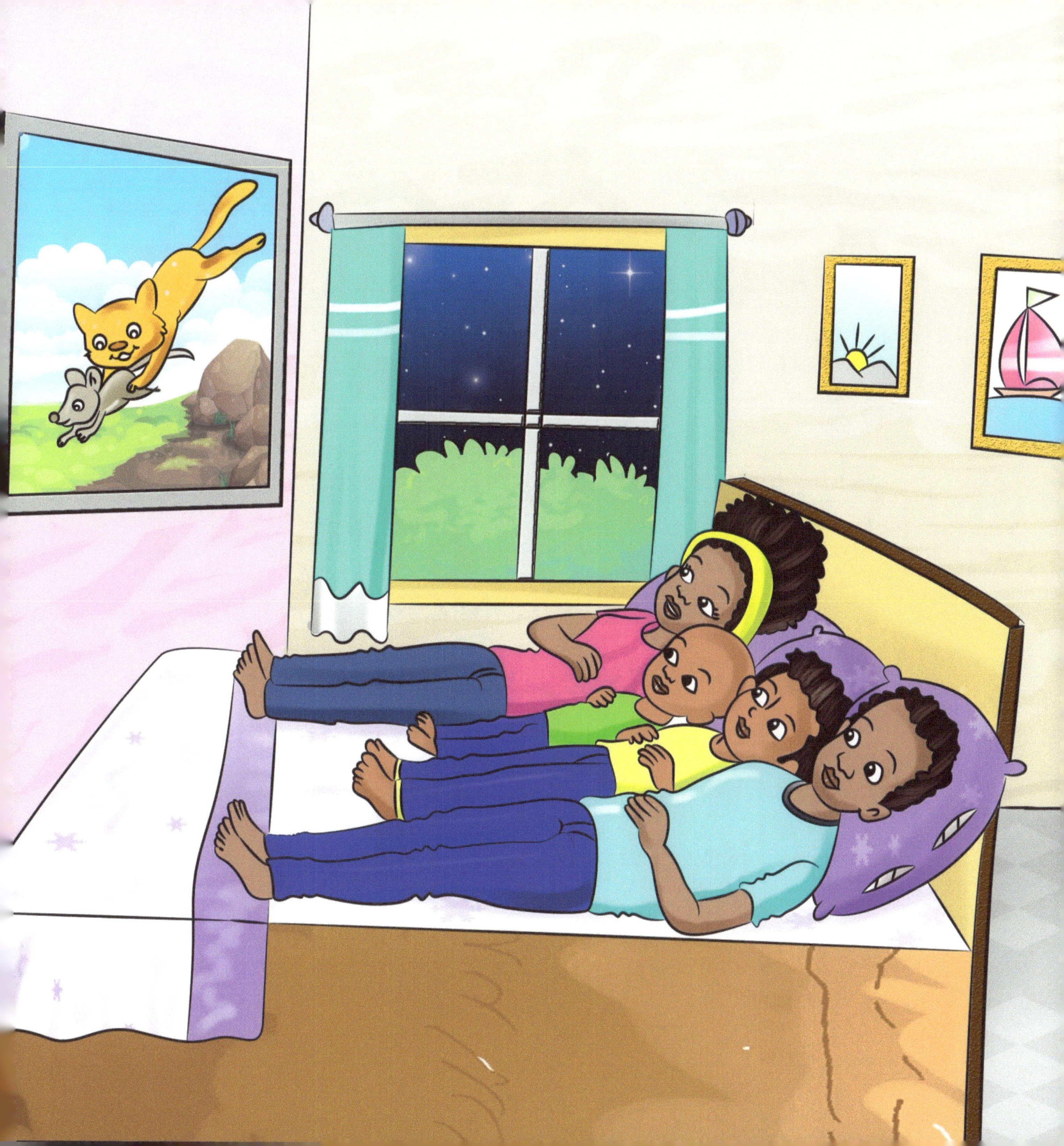

Their parents make sure they have something fun to do everyday for the next few weeks. They paint, have cooking classes, play board games, do scavenger hunts, go on picnics and walks. Their parents also make sure they are able to talk to their family who are far away on FaceTime so they don't feel so disconnected. Camron and Isaiah weren't so bored anymore; though, they did miss playing with their friends.

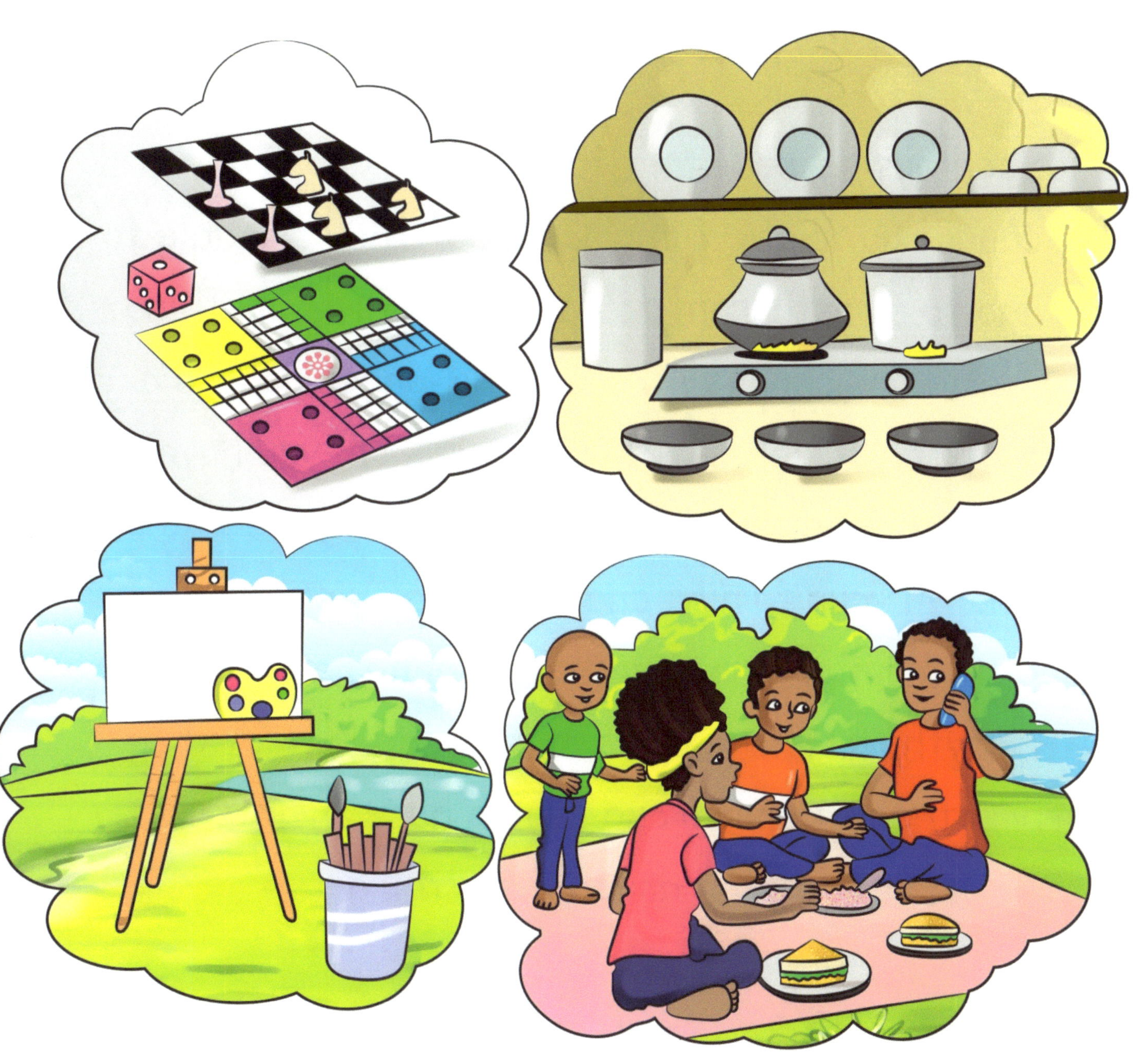

Soon businesses start to open back up. They still cannot go to the fun places, but they are able to go to a restaurant to eat. However, something else has changed. You can no longer go into a store or business without a mask on; you have to stay at least six feet apart from anyone who is not in your family; and their mom kept making them put on hand sanitizer when they touched anything. The masks are hot, and it is hard to breathe in. Camron and Isaiah hate them! COVID has changed everything.

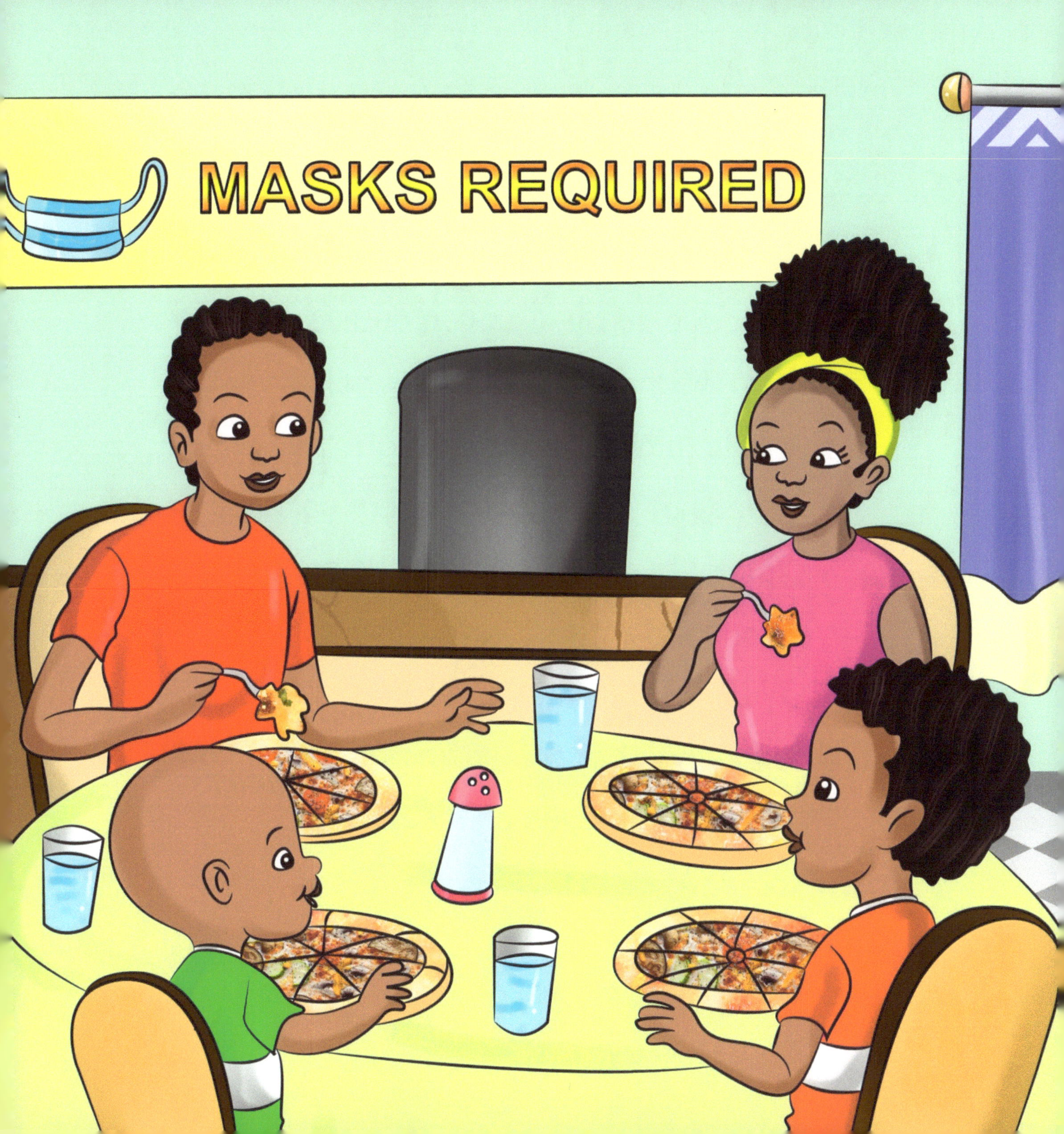

MASKS REQUIRED

As the days go by, Camron and Isaiah get used to wearing the masks when they go into public places. Even though they would rather not wear them, their parents explain: "we wear our masks to keep everyone safe and to stop the spread of COVID." They also make sure to wash their hands before eating or touching their eyes or mouths.

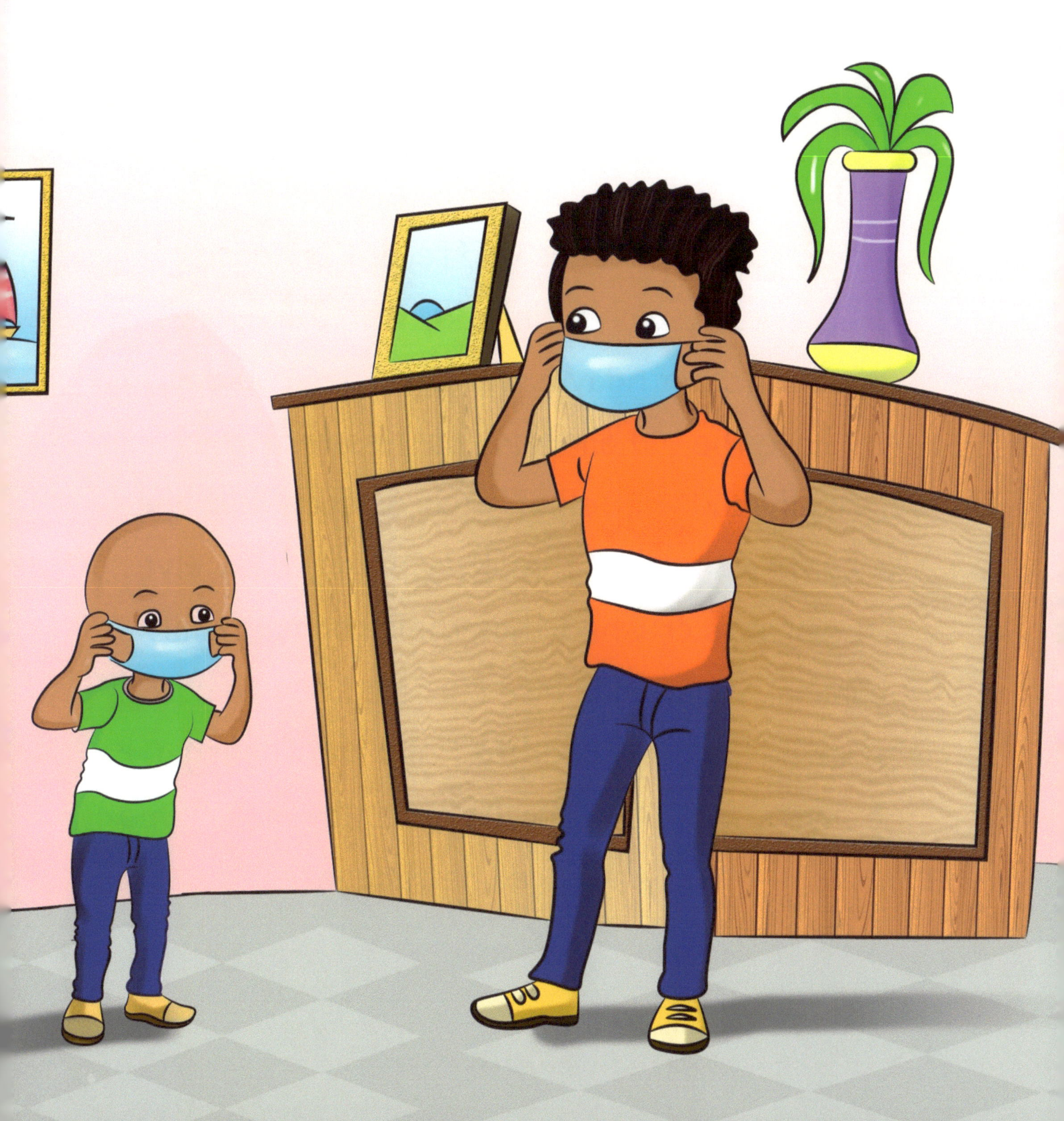

The summer feels so different because of COVID. Isaiah's birthday is in June, and Camron's birthday is in July. They could not have the big birthday parties that they normally had with all of their friends, but their parents make sure that they enjoy themselves. Camron is crushed that their normal family summer vacation is also canceled due to covid, but he is determined to fight the feeling of being upset. 'COVID will not win by making me sad anymore,' he thought.

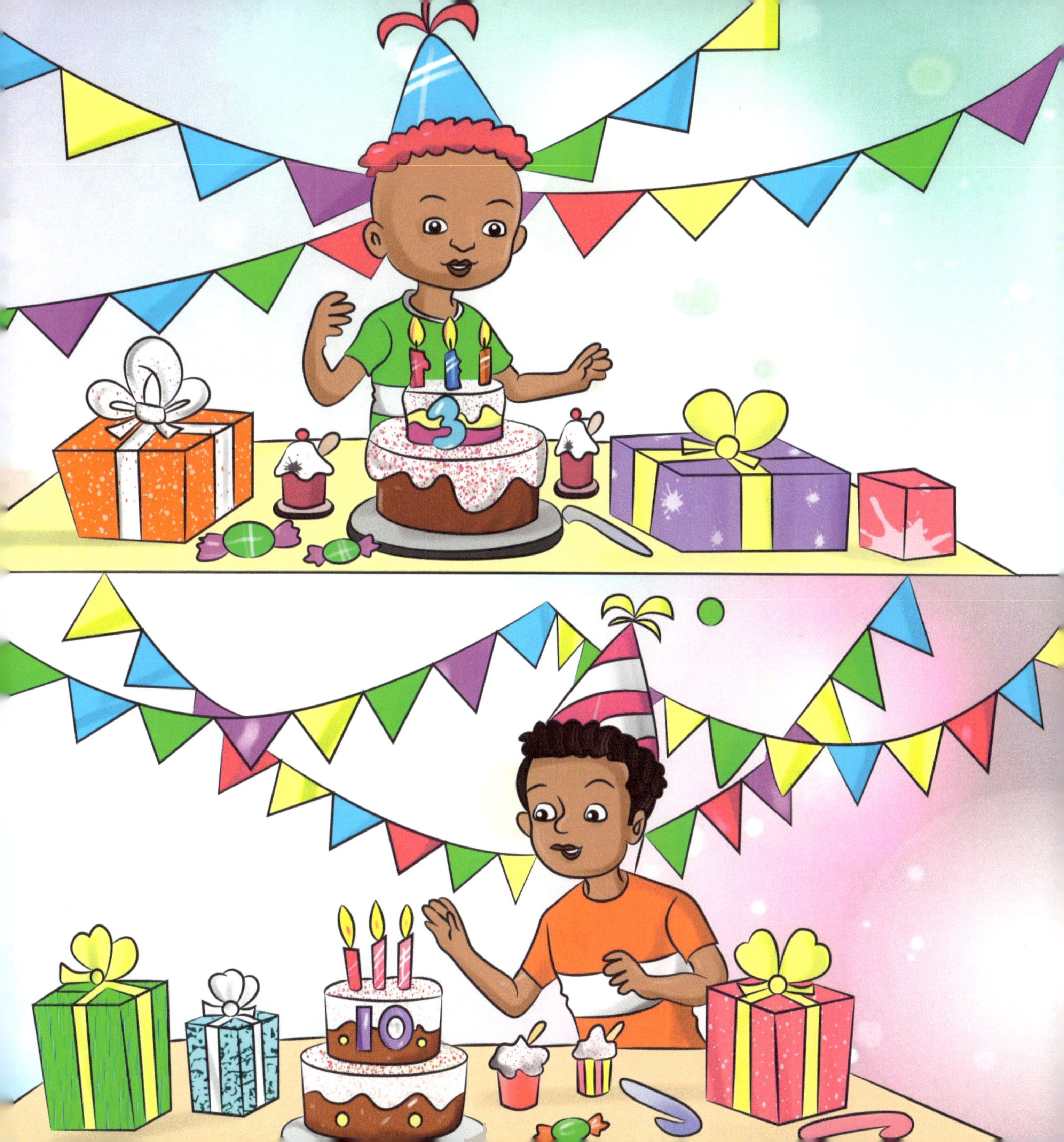

Camron thought about something that he and his family can do together since they can not have a big vacation with their extended family. He asked his dad about a camping trip. "That's a great idea!" Dad said.

A few weeks later their family goes on a camping trip. They have a great time! Even though COVID had come and ruined a lot of things, it did not ruin their family time.

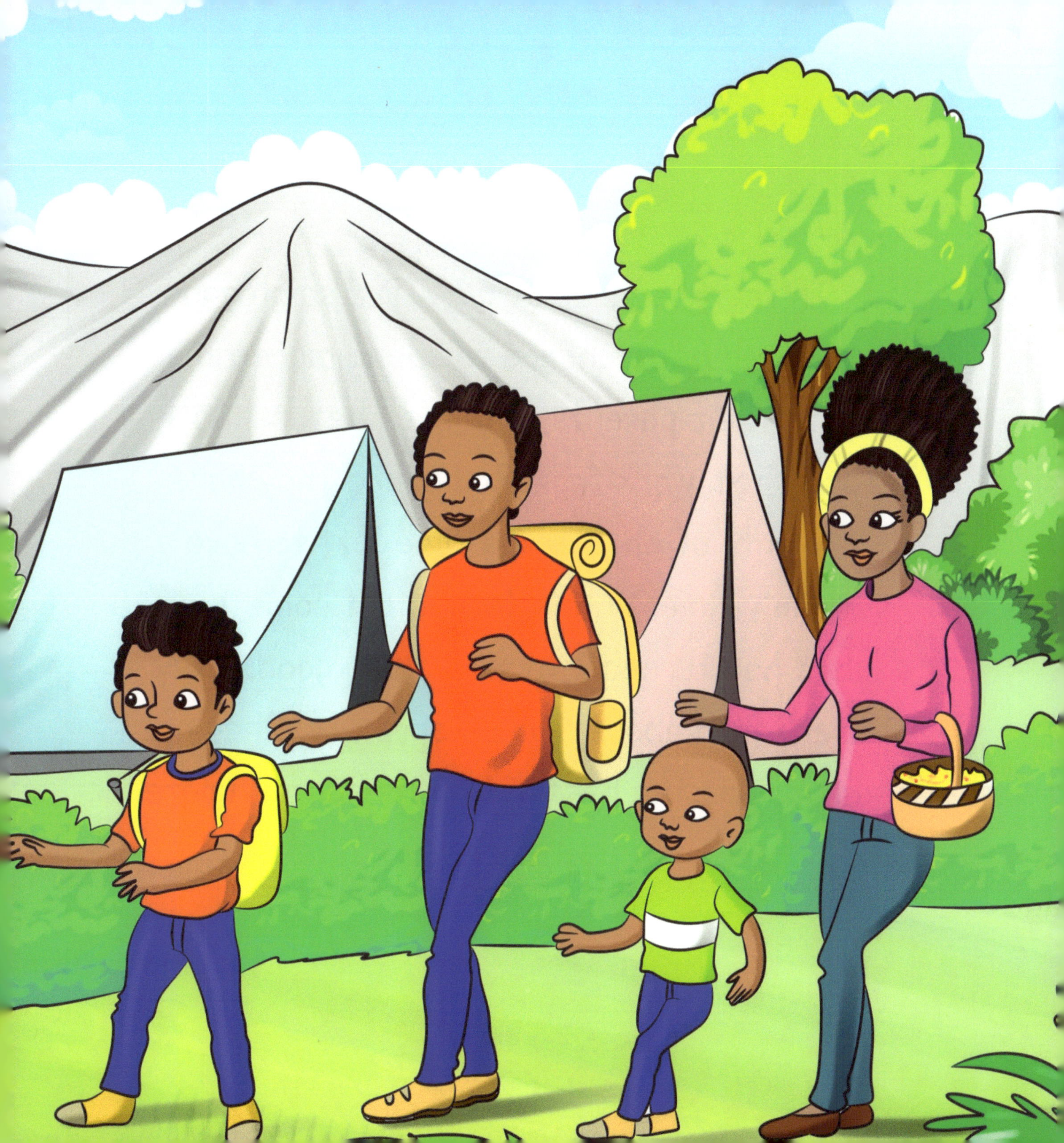

In fact, because of COVID, Isaiah and Camron get a chance to spend more time with their parents than ever before! Both of them work from home, and they have plenty of energy and time left to have family time. What started off something bad had turned into something good. They aren't mad about COVID anymore. They are all making the best out of this unfortunate situation.

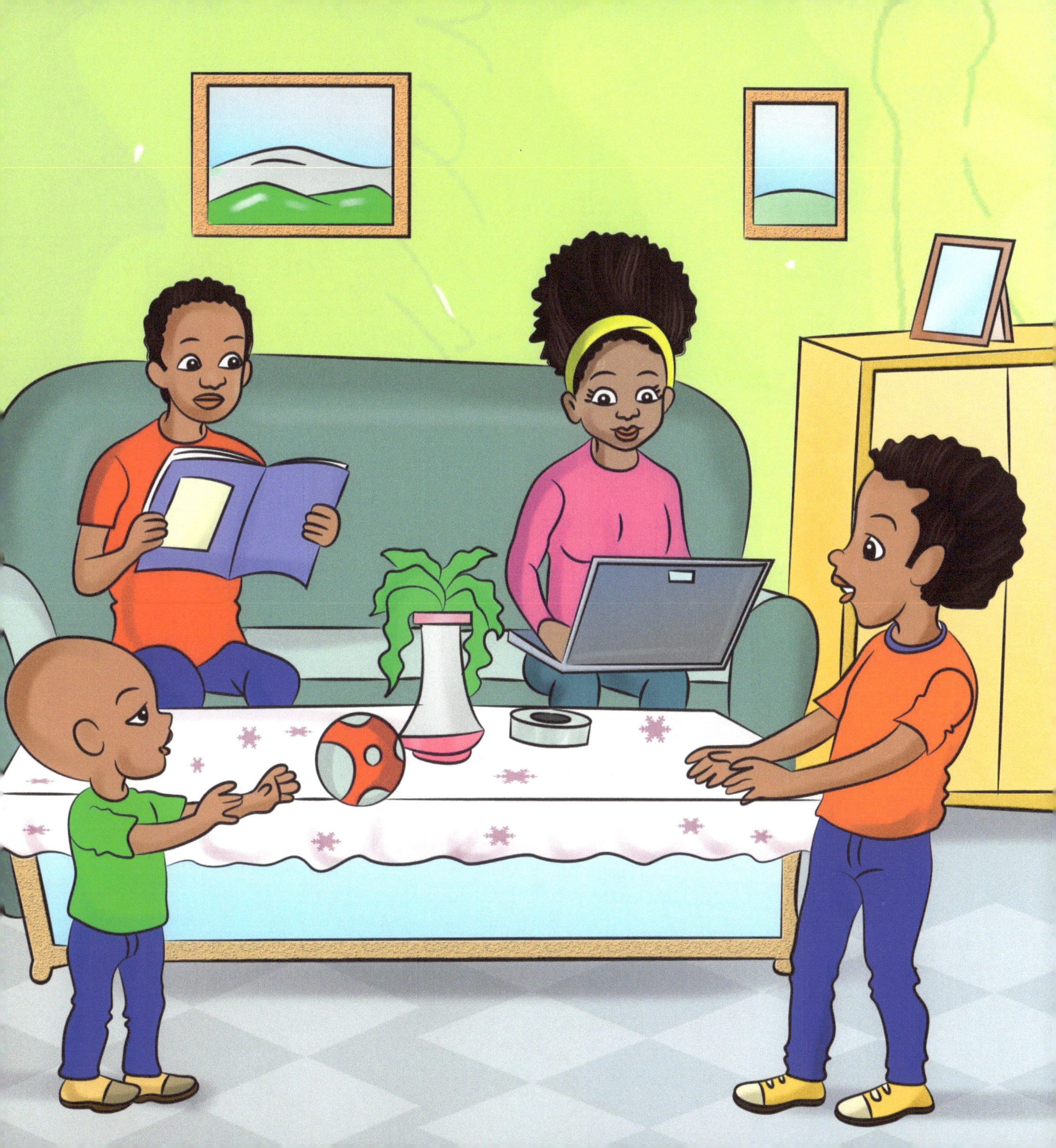

The summer is almost over. Dad returns to work, and Mom begins to plan for the following school year. Camron wonders if they will be returning to school for the fall. His mom says they will not and that they will continue with virtual learning. Camron is a little sad, but he is determined to not let COVID win again. He thinks about all of the positive things. He will still be able to learn and meet with his class online; he won't have to get up super early to catch the bus; and he will still get to spend time with his family. Isaiah is happy that he will not have to go back to daycare just yet.

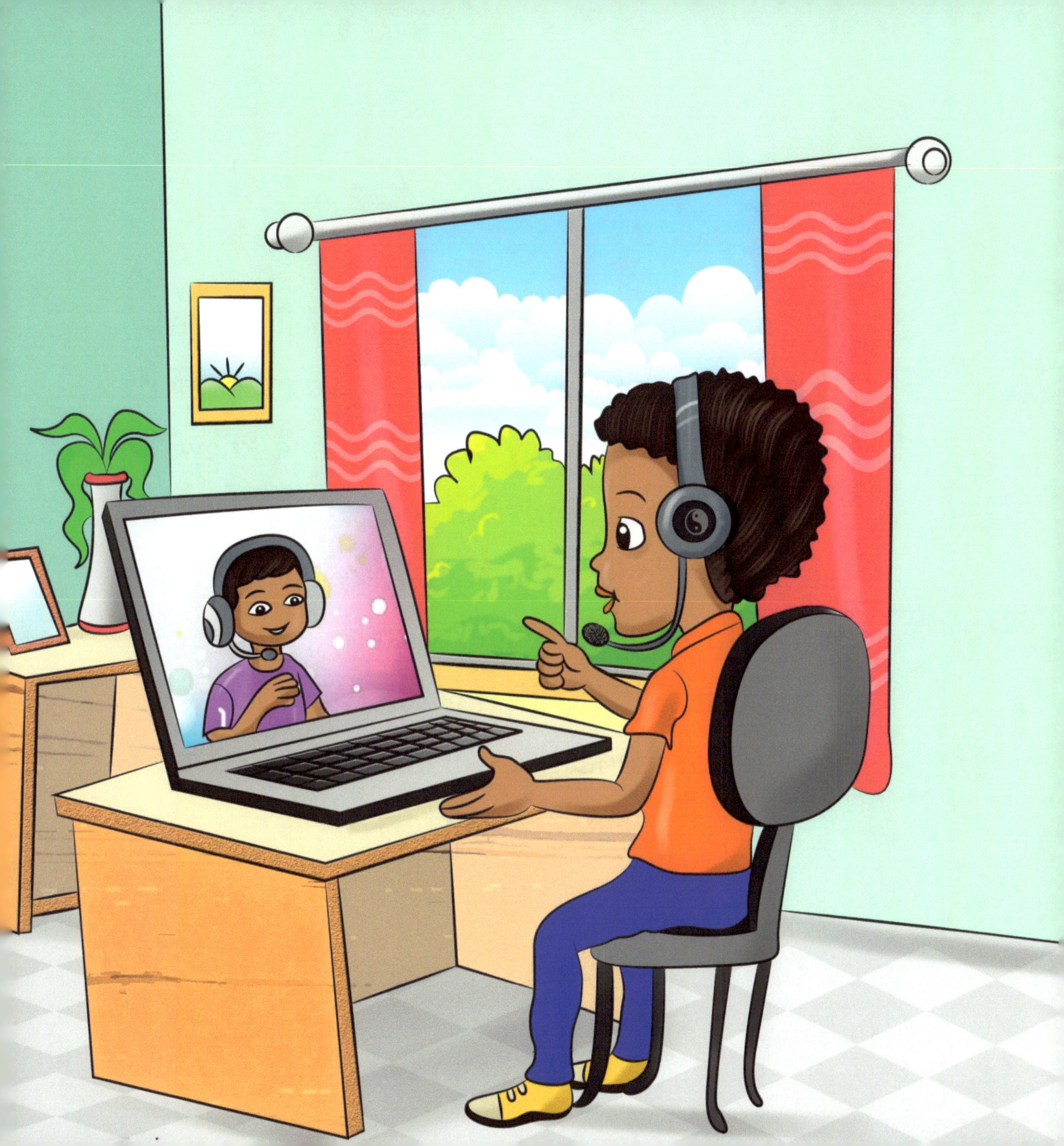

Camron knows things are still not like that last day of school in March. He wonders if it will ever be that way again. No one knows what will happen next. But, one thing Camron and Isaiah do know is that they have their family and their community to help them get through this difficult time! COVID does not win! It just made the world come together and get better!

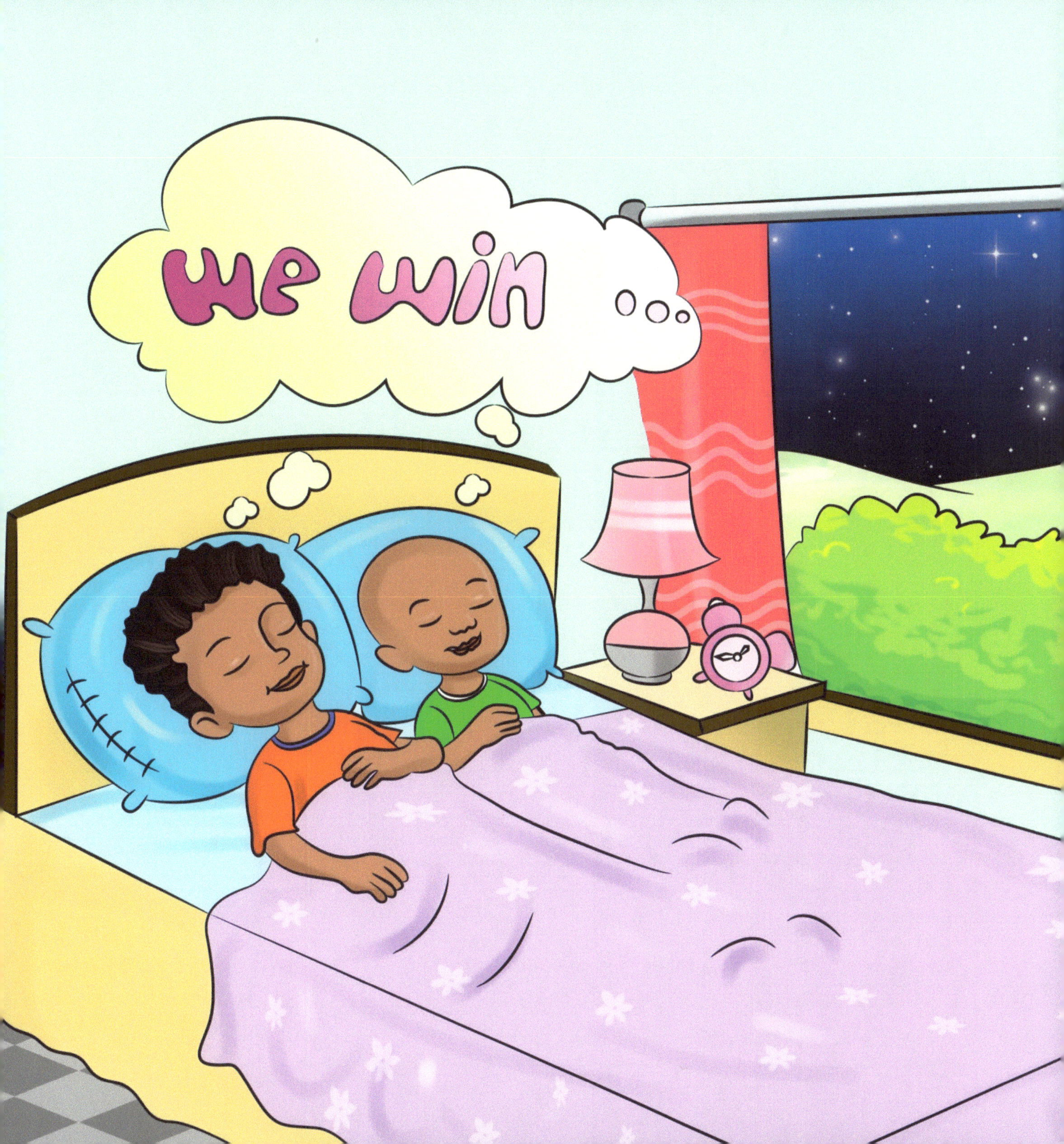
we win ...